Plant-based and Vegan Diets

A Guide for Newbies and The Curious

Peter Weston

A PawPrint Life Upgrades Book

PawPrint Life Upgrades

The PawPrint Life Upgrades series is a series of books commissioned by PawPrint Digital Publishing to help people improve their mental and physical wellbeing, strive for personal success, and realize their life goals.

Acknowledgments

I would like to thank Paul Carlberg BES, and Sabine Pierre for their kind help in preparing this book.

Table of Contents

Introduction

Over the last decade, the mainstream has become aware of what many vegetarians, vegans, and plant-based dieters have known for quite some time: There is a very real health benefit to abstaining from animal products.

Many people also object to the cruel nature of the animal products industries. Traditional farming has been replaced by an increasingly mechanized factory farm method. The quest for increased profits has led to animals being treated as any warehoused inventory item would be treated.

Additionally, the issues that arise from eating meat are often exacerbated by the antibiotics and hormones given to the animals. In the United States, and other countries, animals that are perfectly healthy are given antibiotics as a preventative measure. This leads to a perfect environment to breed drug-resistant diseases, as well as introducing the same antibiotics and hormones into our food chain.

What was considered an odd, extreme diet is increasingly brought to the public eye by various celebrities, pro athletes, and politicians who have switched to plant-based or vegan diets. People now know that you can eschew a meat diet and still succeed in the most competitive arenas.

This short book will provide you with an introduction to living without meat and other animal by-products. By the end of the book, you will know the basics of plant-based diet nutrition, the foods that fulfill those needs, some cooking tips and tricks, and how to stock your pantry and refrigerator with fresh, healthy, wholesome foods. You will understand that what seems like a diet hell to the outsider is in fact a lot easier than you think.

A Note About Your Health

Although almost anyone can abstain from animal food products, any dietary change can not be done lightly. This is especially true if you have any medical condition, known or undiagnosed. Please consult a doctor if you have any health concerns before or after switching your diet.

Chapter 1: What Are Plant-based and Vegan Diets?

Plant-based and vegan seem to be interchangeable terms to many. Both abstain from animal food products. So why are there two different terms? And how are these different from vegetarianism?

Vegetarianism in western society is thought to have originated with the mathematician and philosopher Pythagoras 2,500 years ago. In fact, up until about 200 years ago, vegetarianism was called the "Pythagorean Diet". In India, vegetarianism was advocated by Parshwanatha, a Jain tirthankara 2,800 years ago. Jain vegetarianism forbids eating all animal foods, as well as forbidding eating anything that grows beneath the ground for fear of harming insects and other creatures while digging up the plants. Despite this, most people think of the vegetarian diet as one that forgoes meat, but still includes eggs and dairy products.

The word vegan was coined by Donald Watson of the Vegetarian Society in 1944. He was the secretary for the Leicester branch of the society, and used the word to describe a vegetarian who forgoes all animal-based foods. This was done on ethical grounds. His request to have a non-lacto-vegetarian section added to the Vegetarian Society newsletter was rejected, driving him, and like-minded individuals, to start their own newsletter. He was apparently unhappy with the word vegan, and asked for suggestions of a better descriptive word in the very first newsletter. Vegans not only follow an animal free diet, but also avoid all products that derive from, or harm, animals during production. It is not solely a diet, but an entire ethical and philosophical stance.

The term plant-based diet arose in the 1990's to describe a diet without meat and animal products for the health benefits rather than ethical concerns. A plant-based diet may still include insect products, like honey, where a vegan diet avoids these. Since we are only looking at diet in this book, I will be using the term plant-based diet to include the vegan diet.

Types of Plant-based Diets

In summary, here is a non-exhaustive list of plant-based diets.

1. **Casual/Part-Time/Partial Vegetarians:** There are any number of partial forms of vegetarianism. Some people don't eat mammal-based foods, but are fine with fish and/or birds. Others are vegetarian except for a number of animal products they can't do without. Some are vegetarian except for various holidays or special occasions.

2. **Vegetarians:** Vegetarians forgo all meat, whether it is mammal, bird, or fish. They do, however, eat animal by-products such

as eggs, cheese, and other dairy products.

3. **Plant-based:** The plant-based diet forgoes all animal-based food. The diet excludes animal by-products as well as the meat of all animals. This is done for the health   benefits.

4. **Vegan:** Vegans have a plant-based diet, as well as avoiding all products that harm, or are made from, animals. This is done for ethical   reasons.

5. **Religious diets:** A number of religions have restricted diets. Some demand abstaining from certain types of foods, including some meats, while others demand the utter abstention of all animal-based foods.

Chapter 2: Getting Started

In order to get started, we need a plan. The chapters that follow provide details you need to know to maintain a healthy diet, followed by some of the foods you will need and some cooking tips. Before we do that, however, I am going to provide some advice on how to get started.

- Take it step by step, don't rush. Don't overwhelm yourself.

- Try incorporating foods and recipes into your current diet. Rather than jumping in with both feet, push animal-based products out when you are comfortable with it.

- Look out for plant-based alternatives when shopping. Try different products until you find one you like.

- Many people have had bad experiences with vegan alternatives, and this is mainly due to preparation. Experiment with cooking and preparation until you find what suits you.

- Habits are hard to form and hard to break. Don't make the switch stressful. Have fun with it. You will get there.

Protein

Protein is required for muscle, bone, and organ health. There is a myth that protein is hard to come by without meat. Fortunately, this is a myth. Protein is everywhere. If you were to switch to a lettuce and celery only diet you would be in trouble. If you are worried about your protein intake, or you are a body-builder and need a high protein intake, use nutritional yeast as a supplement.

Iron

Iron is necessary to produce red blood cells that are responsible for transmitting oxygen between organs within the body. While you need to eat iron-rich food items such as broccoli, tofu, beans, and raisins, you should also include food that is rich in vitamin C, such as leafy greens and oranges, as it helps the absorption of iron.

Vitamin B12

Another important component that helps in building red blood cells is vitamin B12. This nutrient is majorly found in seafood, meat, and dairy products, and can therefore be scarce in a plant-based diet. Products such as cereals and soymilk can be substituted for these food items that are rich in vitamin B12. However, you might still need a supplement to fulfill your daily vitamin B12 requirements. Alternatively, nutritional yeast is an excellent source of vitamin B12.

Calcium

We all know that calcium is important to strengthen your bones and teeth. A plant-based diet eliminates all dairy products, so you need other sources. Try adding food items such as broccoli, kale, bok choy, soymilk to your diet. You can also find a few calcium-fortified products in stores. Almonds, lentils, beans, poppy seeds, chia seeds, flaxseeds, edamame, tofu, and figs are all good sources of calcium as well.

Vitamin D

Vitamin D can be obtained from being exposed to sunlight for around 10 minutes daily, depending on your geographic location. Eating calcium-rich food is of no use if you don't consume enough vitamin D, because this is what helps in calcium absorption. Vitamin D deficiency can translate into weaker bones and teeth. A few food items that are rich in vitamin D are mushrooms, cereals, soymilk, and rice milk.

Other Essential Components

Apart from these major components, you also need other essential nutrients such as zinc and omega-3 fatty acids. These are helpful to maintain the health of your immune system, brain, and heart. You can find zinc in nuts, soy products, and beans, while omega-3 fatty acids can be found in flaxseeds, chia seeds, walnuts, and canola oil.

Supplements

If you are new to a plant-based diet, you should consider using supplements that can help you fulfill your daily requirements of vitamin B12, vitamin D, iron, iodine, calcium, the omega-3 fatty acids EPA and DHA, and zinc. While choosing your supplements, don't forget to look for brands that sell vegan products if you want to ensure that there are no animal by-products.

However, you should know that these supplement recommendations do not indicate that your plant-based diet is necessarily inferior or deficient in nutrients. You are just taking additional support for your well-being and ensuring 100% nutrition for optimal health. Ideally, you will eventually get all essential nutrients through your diet. Our digestive system evolved absorbing nutrients in foods, rather than in concentrates. The enzymes that are naturally present along the nutrients help with the absorption. This is referred to as "bioavailability".

Chapter 3: Common Plant-based Diet Foods

This chapter will cover all the major and common plant-based diet items, some of which may be unknown to newbies. While most of you know that a basic shopping list consists of vegetables, nuts, and fruit, let's dig deeper to discover the lesser-known food items and to introduce some versatility into your daily diet.

Make note of these items that are a must-have in your pantry for a basic shopping list at all times.

Nuts and Nut Butter

Nuts are a primary ingredient in almost every plant-based daily diet. Even a single serving of nuts contains a good amount of protein, almost 5 to 12 grams, which can be a great replacement for protein obtained from meat. You can also benefit from the presence of other important nutrients such as magnesium, iron, fiber, vitamin E, and magnesium, among many others. A major benefit of incorporating nuts into your diet is their versatility. You can use them in desserts, as snacks, or consume them in their raw form. If you are fond of nut butter, choose the brands that are organic and natural, as the normal ones are heavily processed and contain additional components such as sugar and oil. Nut butter is also high in protein content and can be a healthy and delicious addition to your daily diet. The most common nuts and nut butters include almond, cashew, and peanuts.

Legumes

Legumes are more of a necessity in a plant-based diet because of their rich protein content. Aside from that, legumes are also rich in iron, which should give you a stronger reason to include them in your diet. You can simply assume that legumes will act as the main meat substitute in any normal daily diet. The common types of legumes consist of beans, chickpeas, and lentils, which are readily available at any store.

Other important nutrients found in legumes are fiber, folate, zinc, manganese, and various antioxidants. However, you should know that legumes also contain antinutrients that slow down the absorption of necessary minerals in your diet. To avoid this issue, you should soak, ferment, or cook your legumes properly—preferably in a pressure cooker—to diminish the effects of these antinutrients. You should also separate legume consumption from meals that are rich in calcium, as calcium decreases the absorption of iron. You can, however, consume legumes with food items that are rich in vitamin C, as it will increase iron absorption.

Meat Substitutes

The most common types of meat substitutes include items made from soybeans such as tofu and tempeh. Apart from legumes, most plant-based diets include these two items as a source of protein. A 100-gram portion of tofu or tempeh contains 16 to 19 grams of protein, which is a high amount compared to other food sources. Tofu is made from soybean curds and tempeh is made by fermenting soybeans for a certain period of time. You can prepare both these items by grilling or sautéing, which makes them fantastic replacements for eggs and fish in practically any recipe. Since soybeans also contain a small amount of antinutrients, the fermentation process is helpful in reducing their quantity and increasing the production of vitamin B12. Another commonly used alternative for meat is seitan, which is rich in selenium, protein (25 grams per serving of 100 grams), calcium, iron, and phosphorus. Seitan is wheat flour gluten which can be bought as "wheat meat" or in powdered form.

Fruits and Vegetables

Fruits and vegetables are, undoubtedly, the most common food items in every plant-based diet. These are nutrient-dense and provide a number of health benefits. Also, a few vegetables and fruits can be great substitutes for meat to add texture, color, and flavor to various dishes. Green leafy vegetables are rich in iron and calcium content and should definitely take up a major part of your diet. You should also add the following veggies to your diet: cauliflower, eggplant, bok choy, spinach, mustard greens, kale, and watercress, among many others. Fruits such as apples, bananas, oranges, pomegranates, and berries should be purchased on a regular basis. These ingredients can make great substitutes for meat-based and dairy-based dishes:

- Use blended bananas to make frozen desserts with a consistency similar to ice cream.
- Use blended cauliflower as a base for pizza crust.
- Make sandwiches and stir-fries with jackfruits.
- Use mushrooms and eggplants for a great texture in any dish.

Various Types of Seeds

You might have heard about the use of chia seeds and flaxseeds in several weight-loss meal plans. Not only are these healthy, but they're also a great addition to your plant-based diet. Put chia seeds, flaxseeds, and hemp seeds on your list because these are amazing sources of protein, as well as omega-3 and omega-6 fatty acids. They can help to combat various health issues such as skin conditions, inflammation, menopause, and premenstrual syndrome (PMS). An important component known as the alpha-linolenic acid (ALA) is found in abundance in chia seeds and flaxseeds, which gets converted into two other important components known as eicosapentaenoic acid (EPA) and docosahexaenoic acid (DHA). These are usually found in fish and are helpful to improve our nervous system, reducing inflammation, and boosting mental health. This is why it is necessary to add these seeds to your diet.

Plant-Based Dairy Alternatives

Since all dairy products come from animals, they are eliminated from every plant-based diet. As we all know, calcium is necessary to build healthy bones and teeth, and its deficiency can result in weaker bone health and cause severe complications in the long run. To minimize this risk, you should consume calcium-rich, non-dairy food items that can make up for the daily calcium requirements. You should look for fortified plant-based milk and yogurt products that are abundant in calcium and vitamin D (to help your body absorb the calcium). A few brands sell dairy alternative products add vitamin D and vitamin B12 to their formulas, which can be extremely useful. Other plant-based dairy alternatives include milk made from soy, hemp, cashews, or milk and yogurt made from coconut, rice, oats, and almonds. Try to go for the unsweetened versions to lower your daily sugar intake.

Nutritional Yeast

Nutritional yeast is made from Saccharomyces cerevisiae (beer yeast). It is deactivated and can be found in almost any grocery store. This is a great source of vitamin B12, protein, fiber, and other essential nutrients such as copper, manganese, zinc, and magnesium. Nutritional yeast is usually found in the form of flakes or yellow powder. Not many people know about the benefits and use of nutritional yeast to fulfill daily vitamin B12 requirements. With 7 grams of fiber and 14 grams of protein present in one ounce of nutritional yeast, this ingredient is a great addition to your shopping list. However, be sure to not buy this fortified nutritional yeast in clear bags, as the vitamin B12 content might degrade when exposed to light. Deactivated beer yeast can be bought as well. It is a non-fortified powder which contains the nutrients and protein you find in meat, and is cheaper than nutritional yeast. Some nutritional yeast products were formulated in the days of vitamin "megadosing" and have not been updated to reflect our current understanding of vitamin absorption. If a product has 800 - 1000% of the recommended daily intake, you should probably avoid it.

Cereals and Whole Grains

Whether you follow a vegetarian, plant-based, or traditional diet, cereals and whole grains are probably common ingredients in your household. These are rich in essential nutrients such as fiber, complex carbs, vitamins B6 & B12, zinc, phosphorus, iron, and magnesium, among others. The term 'pseudo-cereals' is very common in the plant-based diet world. It refers to a 'higher' form of cereals that can substitute common grains such as wheat and rice. These include teff, buckwheat, quinoa, and amaranth. They are not only rich in protein but add more taste and texture to every dish. One cup of cooked teff contains 10 to 11 grams of protein, whereas one cup of cooked quinoa or amaranth contains around 9 grams of protein.

These protein-rich pseudo-cereals should be substituted for normal grains as much as possible. The only downsides to these are that they can be a bit on the pricier side, and they also contain traces of antinutrients. However, better cooking techniques and sprouting can reduce the effect of these antinutrients.

Fermented and Sprouted Plant-Based Food

As we already know by now, most plant-based food items contain a few traces of antinutrients that block the absorption of necessary minerals in your body. You can solve this issue, for the most part, by sprouting or fermenting these plant-based products. Not only do these processes help to reduce the impact of antinutrients but they also improve the protein quality. You can find a number of pre-fermented products in stores such as kimchi, kombucha, miso, tempeh, Ezekiel bread, natto, pickles, and sauerkraut. Some of these can be difficult to find at times because they are mostly available in regional stores. If you want to benefit from sprouting and fermentation, you can practice it at home with grains. These fermented food products contain probiotic bacteria and vitamin K2, which boost the immune system and improve bone health, respectively. They can also protect you from major health issues such as heart disease and cancer.

Seaweed

Seaweed is rich in DHA, protein, iodine, and various minerals such as manganese, magnesium, riboflavin, potassium, and antioxidants. DHA is a type of fatty acid and is essential for your body. Also, seaweed is so high in iodine content that all plant-based diets should include it. It boosts your metabolism and enhances the functioning of the thyroid gland. Among the various types of edible seaweed and algae available today, kelp is comparatively high in iodine content. Other types of seaweed include spirulina and chlorella. Seaweed is a great source of antioxidants as well, which means it can help to release harmful toxins from your body. With 8 grams of protein present in a serving of two tablespoons, seaweed forms another prime ingredient on your list.

Summary

To sum it up, here is a list of items to keep an eye out for:

- **Fruit (Fresh):** Apples, bananas, watermelons, dates, pomegranates, kiwis, figs, berries (raspberries, strawberries, blueberries), citrus fruits (lemons, oranges, grapefruits, clementine and limes), stone fruits (cherries, peaches, nectarines, plums), melons (honeydew and cantaloupe), and tropical or seasonal fruits (pineapples, mangoes, jackfruit, durian, dragon fruit, papaya, lychee, passion fruit).

- **Fruit (Frozen):** Cherries, mangoes, pineapples, peaches, mixed fruits, berries (strawberries, blueberries, blackberries, raspberries).

- **Dried Fruit:** Apricots, mangoes, raisins, apples, cherries, figs, cranberries, goji berries, mulberries, dates.

- **Vegetables (Fresh):** Green leafy vegetables (spinach, arugula, kale, collard greens), cabbage (of all types), lettuce (of all types), cauliflower, zucchini, cucumber, tomato, carrot, artichoke, bell pepper, beet, asparagus, broccoli, potato, turnip, yam, celery, avocado, hot pepper, garlic, eggplant, ginger, onion, mushroom, squash, green beans, and peas.

- **Vegetables (Canned or Frozen):** Tomato paste and puree, corn, pumpkin, peas, artichoke, broccoli, mixed veggies, brussels sprouts, green beans, and butternut squash.

- **Legumes:** Kidney beans, black-eyed beans, white kidney beans, lentils, pinto beans, split peas, and navy beans (among many other types).

- **Whole Grains and Related Products:**

Brown or wild rice, millet, rolled or steel-cut oats, farro, quinoa, amaranth, buckwheat, barley, freekeh, teff, whole-grain bread, whole-grain pasta, whole-grain flours, and rice cakes.

- **Dairy Alternatives:** Non-dairy milk (soy, almond, oat, rice, coconut, cashew, or hemp), yogurt (almond, coconut, cashew), and cashew cheese.

- **Nuts and Seeds:** Walnuts, cashew nuts, almonds, pecans, pine nuts, hazelnuts, pistachios, sunflower seeds, chia seeds, hemp seeds, flaxseeds, sesame seeds, and pumpkin seeds. You can also buy respective nut and seed butters if available. Tahini is available as a spread or sauce made from sesame seeds.

These are the basic 'main' ingredients that should be on your list. Apart from these, you should consider buying soy products, herbs and spices, condiments, sweeteners and various other plant-based items that are easily available.

Chapter 4: Food Recipes

Plant-based diet cooking may be new to you, but with practice you will be making delicious meals in no time. Here are a few ideas just to inspire you:

Crispy Tofu and Quinoa

Prep time: 10 mins

Cooking time: 25 mins

Total time: 35 mins

Ingredients:

15 ounces of tofu

1 cup of cooked quinoa

½ cup of thinly sliced red onion

¼ cup of rice wine vinegar

¼ cup of sweet chili sauce

3 tbsp. of corn-flour (cornstarch)

1 tbsp of halved and roasted cashews

1 cup of chopped and deseeded cucumber

Vegetable oil for frying

Olive oil, parsley, and salt for seasoning

Directions:

Cut the tofu in cubes and pat them dry with paper towels, making sure you get rid of as much moisture as possible. Coat them with corn-flour and fry them until they are crispy. Mix vinegar, olive oil, chili sauce, and some salt in a bowl. Add this mixture to the red onion and cucumber slices and mix well.

Serve the quinoa in a bowl along with some parsley, roasted cashews, prepared salad, and tofu.

Vegan Crab Cakes

Prep time: 15 mins

Cooking time: 15 mins

Chilling time: 1 hour

Total time: 90 mins

Ingredients:

25 ounces of jackfruit (fresh or canned)

1 tsp of mustard powder

2 tbsp of flaxseeds

1 tsp of Worcestershire sauce (vegan)

1 tbsp of lemon juice

½ tsp of garlic powder

½ tsp of black pepper powder

¼ cup of chopped cilantro

3 tbsp of chopped chives

1 cup of breadcrumbs

Directions:

Grind the flaxseeds and mix it with 90 ml of water. Let this mixture sit for 10 mins. Meanwhile, mix the mustard powder in a teaspoon of water. Add the lemon juice, Worcestershire sauce, and mustard, mixing them well. Pat dry the jackfruit to avoid sogginess and chop it into lumps that resemble crab meat. Now, add the jackfruit, chives, cilantro, seasonings and the flaxseed mixture to the breadcrumbs. Shape them into cubes and refrigerate them for an hour.

You can either bake or fry these cakes:

- Preheat the oven to 375 degrees and bake them for 10 minutes on each side.

- Shallow-fry them in 2 tablespoons of oil and cook them for 5 minutes on each side until they are golden brown. Serve with sriracha and lemon.

Butternut Squash Chipotle

Preparation time: 20 mins

Cooking time: 1 hour

Total time: 80 mins

Ingredients:

1 ½ pounds of peeled, chopped, and cubed butternut squash

2 chopped bell peppers (preferably red)

1 medium chopped red onion

4 cloves of garlic, minced

1 bay leaf

¼ tsp of cinnamon powder

1 tsp of chili powder

1 tsp of cumin powder

½ tbsp of chipotle pepper (chopped)

15 ounces of black beans, cooked

14 ounces of vegetable broth

14 ounces of tomatoes, diced

2 cups of crumbled tortilla chips

2 diced avocados

¼ tbsp of cilantro

Directions:

Sauté the bell peppers, butternut squash, and onions in olive oil and stir occasionally until the onions are translucent. Add the minced garlic, cumin, cinnamon, chipotle pepper, bay leaf, tomatoes, broth, and black beans. Let it come to the boil, then cover and let simmer for about an hour. Once the squash is nice and tender, season with chili and salt.

Garnish it with cilantro and serve with diced avocados and tortilla chips.

Dark Chocolate Tofu "Cheesecake"

Preparation time: 20 mins

Cooking time: 10 mins

Total time: 30 mins

Ingredients:

For the crust:

1 cup of pretzels

½ cup of peanut butter

2 tbsp of coconut oil (melt it if solid)

1 tbsp of maple syrup

For the topping:

1 pound of tofu

1 tsp of vanilla extract

2 tbsp of coffee

12 ounces of dark chocolate

Directions:

Blend the pretzels in a food processor for a minute or two until they form crumbs. Add maple syrup, peanut butter, and coconut oil and blend for a few seconds. Transfer this mixture to a pan and spread it evenly. Preheat the oven to 350 degrees and bake for 10 minutes. Remove the pan and let it cool.

To make the filling, melt the chocolate over low heat until no lumps are visible. Place the tofu, maple syrup, vanilla extract, and melted chocolate in a food processor and blend it until smooth and creamy. You can add more maple syrup if you want the filling to be sweeter. Now, pour this mixture on the crust, spread evenly, and refrigerate overnight to let the filling set.

Serve the cake with some coconut whipped cream and berries.

Some Extra Tips

Recipes can be adapted to replace meat and animal by-products. Here are a couple of tips to get you started.

Eggs and Egg Whites

Chia seeds can substitute for eggs where the egg is

used as a binder. A ratio of 1:3 with water will do the trick. Lightly grind the seed in a coffee grinder or with a pestle and mortar. Mix the ground chia seed with water and let sit for five minutes for it to set. Use in place of eggs in your recipe.

As an extra extra tip, ground chia seed is also very good for making a quick all natural jam. Buy frozen berries and let them thaw almost all the way. You can also freeze fresh berries and thaw. The frozen berries release moisture as they complete the thaw, helping with the gelling process. The ratio should be two cups of fruit with two tablespoons of chia seed. Mash the mostly thawed fruit in a blender and then stir in the chia seed and an equal amount of lemon or apple juice. Let sit for half-an-hour, stirring once. Put in a jar and refrigerate.

This will not have the Jello like consistency of store bought jam, but it does very nicely on toast, hot cereals, or plant-based yogurt. It adds the benefit of having protein, added calcium, and omega-3.

Ground Beef or Pork

Tofu can substitute for ground beef or pork in chilis, stews, stir fries and sloppy joes. Use a quarter brick of extra-firm tofu for each person being served. Cut each quarter into three or four slices, place flat with paper-towel on the top and bottom. Place a frying pan or some other heavy item on top for about fifteen minutes to squeeze out the moisture. Crumble the tofu by rolling between your palms and pinching apart. Heat a couple of tablespoons of canola oil in a frying pan on medium heat. When hot, add the tofu and leave for a couple of minutes. Stir and leave again for a couple of minutes. Stir in an appropriate sauce for your recipe. If you are making a stir fry, add your vegetables with the sauce. Cook over medium heat for an additional ten minutes, stirring once or twice. In that time, the sauce will caramelize on the tofu and make a slightly crunchy outer coating.

Summary

These are just a few plant-based recipe ideas to give you a kick-start and add some excitement to your routine. A lot of people that want to switch to a plant-based diet are afraid of taking the first step toward this lifestyle because they think the meal options would be limited. I hope that this chapter has inspired you to make delicious and event-worthy recipes that are just as decadent as 'normal' meals. Just start with the basics, and experiment with recipes by adding a personal touch.

Chapter 5: How to Maintain a Plant-based Diet

Going meat free can be extremely difficult for some people. Starting it is easy but staying consistent is difficult. Follow these tips to maintain a plant-based diet.

Plan Ahead

Prepare a list of ingredients and recipes ahead of time and cook your meals accordingly. You need to stick to your meal plan in order to stick to a diet. You can either keep a journal or hang a weekly meal plan in your kitchen where it will be visible all the time, like your fridge. To make it easier, you can meal-prep and cook for the next few days. This way, you'll save a lot of time, won't waste food, and you'll get to stick to your diet even when you're in a rush.

Stock Up

This point is somewhat connected to the above-mentioned tip. If you have enough food at home, you probably won't be tempted to order something else or cook something that you are not supposed to eat. Stock up on food items that are suitable for a plant-based diet, and cook only with those ingredients. Keep them in bulk in order not to get distracted. Also, always go grocery shopping with a full stomach, or at least after a meal or a snack. This will keep you motivated to stick to your plan.

Do Not Stay Hungry for Long

While you are planning your meals and stocking up on ingredients, make sure that you also eat them on time. Plan your daily schedule and include specific meal timings. More importantly, stick to those. Keep all the meals and snacks prepared so you are not tempted to indulge. It will be a bit difficult at the beginning, but you will slowly adjust to the routine.

Experiment with New Recipes

One reason that you might give up easily is monotony. If you keep on eating the same dishes and using the same ingredients to cook on a daily basis, you will soon get bored. Since you already know about the myriad of ingredients that can be included in a plant-based diet, try adding variety to your pantry and experiment with new recipes. This will keep you creative and consistent.

Remember Why You Started It

The key is to stay motivated.You cannot cheat out of temptation or turn to your favorite food 'just for one day.' You need to reflect on the reason why you started and what motivated you to go on a plant-based diet. The main reason that motivated you was probably the empathy you felt toward animals, the need for a healthier lifestyle, or both. Remember this reason whenever you are tempted to go back to a traditional diet and keep a positive attitude at all times.

By following these tips, you will not only follow a consistent lifestyle but also maintain a healthy body. Planning ahead and eating on time will give you more control over your daily life, as well.

Lastly, remember that a major change in diet can exacerbate medical conditions, even if you don't know you have any. If you have any concerns, see your medical doctor before, during, or after the change if anything seems wrong.

Conclusion

After going through these chapters, you must realize by now that a plant-based diet is not as 'extreme' as many claim. You just need the right information and a little bit of motivation to permanently incorporate a plant-based diet into your lifestyle. After you get a better understanding of the basics such as nutrition, food sources, and meal preparation, you need to make a plan and stick to it. More importantly, pay maximum attention to your nutrition. No diet would be worth following if you couldn't provide your body with enough nutrition. You can switch to healthier food options and take help from supplements, as we've discussed throughout the guide.

To sum it up, here are a few more tips and factors that are important while transitioning into a plant-based diet:

- Add as many portions of fruit and vegetables as you can to your daily diet (a minimum of 5 portions are recommended).

- Always store basic plant-based dairy alternatives such as soymilk and soy yogurt. You can both consume these directly and use them as ingredients while experimenting with recipes.

- Use wheat, rice, potatoes, and pasta as the base of your meals when you are in a hurry.

- Always choose organic and unsaturated spreads and oils for better health.

- Always consult with your medical doctor before using supplements. While buying, check the labels for a 'vegan' sign. Remember that a plant-based diet and vegan diet are essentially the same. The differences are what you do beyond your diet.

- Stay hydrated. If you had a low fibre intake before switching, this is especially important.

- Try to combine a variety of ingredients on your plate—preferably of all colors—to gain maximum nutritional benefits.

- There are a number of excellent nutrition monitoring and diet tracking apps available to help. Remember that counting calories is not what you're looking for. You want to track your vitamin and nutrient intake.

I hope that this guide has inspired you to make some changes in your own life and motivated you to begin your journey as soon as possible. Good luck!

www.ingramcontent.com/pod-product-compliance
Lightning Source LLC
Chambersburg PA
CBHW050748250726
48662CB00005B/2092